# My Complete Dash Diet Cooking Guide

## A Quick and Easy Collection of Dash Diet Recipes

Eleonore Barlow

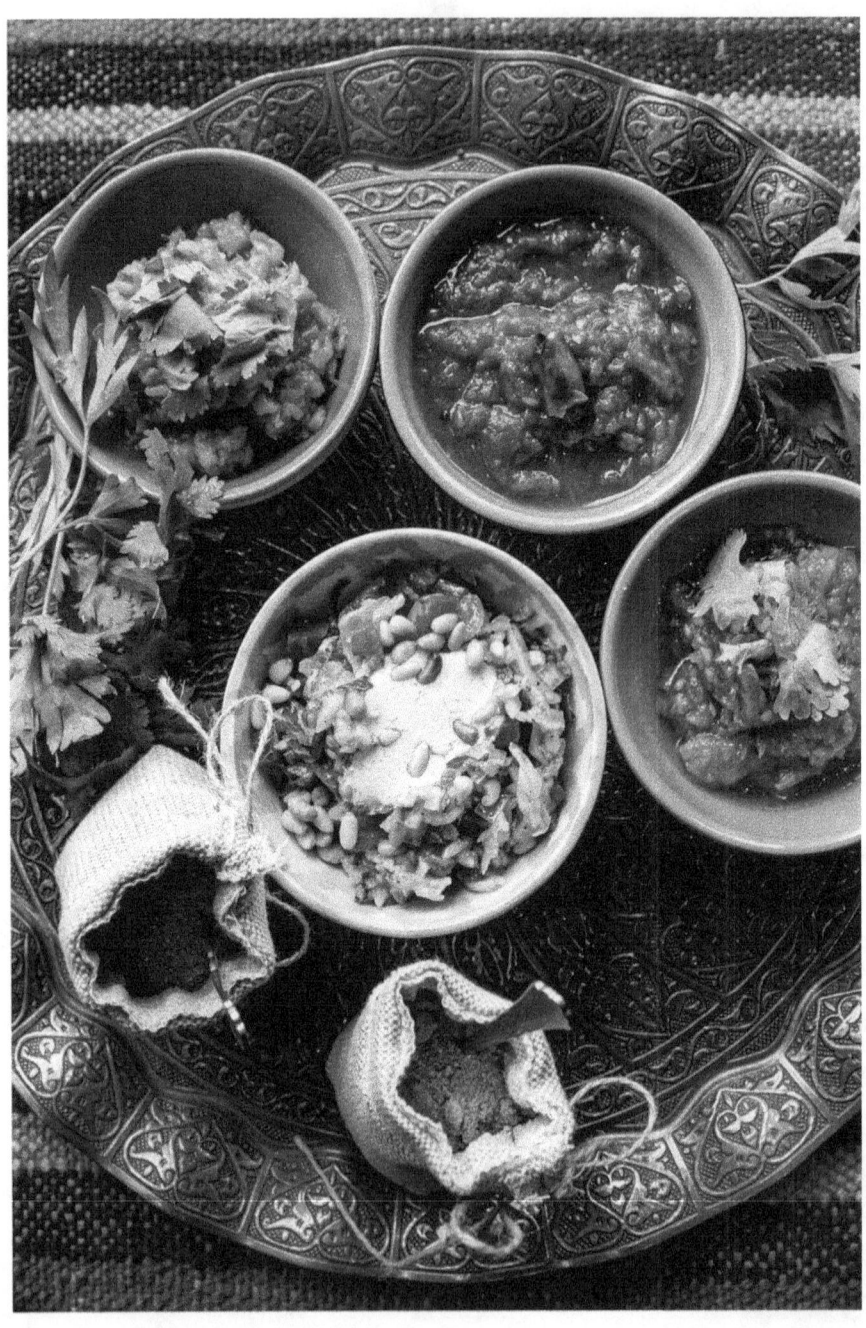

© Copyright 2021 - All rights reserved.

The content contained within this book may not be reproduced, duplicated or transmitted without direct written permission from the author or the publisher.
Under no circumstances will any blame or legal responsibility be held against the publisher, or author, for any damages, reparation, or monetary loss due to the information contained within this book. Either directly or indirectly.

**Legal Notice:**
This book is copyright protected. This book is only for personal use. You cannot amend, distribute, sell, use, quote or paraphrase any part, or the content within this book, without the consent of the author or publisher.

**Disclaimer Notice:**
Please note the information contained within this document is for educational and entertainment purposes only. All effort has been executed to present accurate, up to date, and reliable, complete information. No warranties of any kind are declared or implied. Readers acknowledge that the author is not engaging in the rendering of legal, financial, medical or professional advice. The content within this book has been derived from various sources. Please consult a licensed professional before attempting any techniques outlined in this book.
By reading this document, the reader agrees that under no circumstances is the author responsible for any losses, direct or indirect, which are incurred as a result of the use of information contained within this document, including, but not limited to, — errors, omissions, or inaccuracies.

# Table of Contents

| | |
|---|---:|
| Vanilla Sweet Potato Porridge | 6 |
| A Nice German Oatmeal | 8 |
| Very Nutty Banana Oatmeal | 10 |
| Cool Coconut Flatbread | 12 |
| Perfect Homemade Pickled Ginger Gari | 14 |
| Avocado and Blueberry Medley | 16 |
| Healthy Zucchini Stir Fry | 18 |
| Greek Lemon Chicken Bowl | 20 |
| Chilled Chicken, Artichoke and Zucchini Platter | 22 |
| Chicken and Carrot Stew | 24 |
| Tasty Spinach Pie | 26 |
| Mesmerizing Carrot and Pineapple Mix | 28 |
| Ethiopian Cabbage Delight | 30 |
| The Vegan Lovers Refried Beans | 32 |
| Cool Apple and Carrot Harmony | 34 |
| Mac and Chokes | 36 |
| Bay Scallop Chowder | 39 |
| Salmon and Vegetable Soup | 41 |
| Garlic Tomato Soup | 43 |
| Melon Soup | 45 |
| Spring Salad | 46 |
| Hearty Orange and Onion Salad | 48 |
| Ground Beef Bell Peppers | 50 |
| Ecstatic "Foiled" Fish | 52 |
| Brazilian Shrimp Stew | 54 |
| Inspiring Cajun Snow Crab | 56 |

| | |
|---|---|
| GRILLED LIME SHRIMP | 58 |
| CALAMARI CITRUS | 61 |
| BAKED CHICKEN | 63 |
| ORANGE CHICKEN AND BROCCOLI STIR-FRY | 65 |
| MEDITERRANEAN LEMON CHICKEN AND POTATOES | 67 |
| TANDOORI CHICKEN | 69 |
| GRILLED CHICKEN SALAD | 72 |
| HEARTY CASHEW AND ALMOND BUTTER | 74 |
| RED COLESLAW | 76 |
| AVOCADO MAYO MEDLEY | 78 |
| AMAZING GARLIC AIOLI | 80 |
| EASY SEED CRACKERS | 82 |
| HEARTY ALMOND CRACKERS | 84 |
| BLACK BEAN SALSA | 86 |
| DELISH PINEAPPLE AND COCONUT MILK SMOOTHIE | 88 |
| THE MINTY REFRESHER | 89 |
| THE "UPBEAT" STRAWBERRY AND CLEMENTINE GLASS | 91 |
| CABBAGE AND COCONUT CHIA SMOOTHIE | 93 |
| THE CHERRY BEET DELIGHT | 95 |
| SATISFYING HONEY AND COCONUT PORRIDGE | 97 |
| PURE MAPLE GLAZED CARROTS | 99 |
| GINGER AND ORANGE "BEETS" | 101 |
| PINEAPPLE RICE | 103 |
| CREATIVE LEMON AND BROCCOLI DISH | 105 |

# Vanilla Sweet Potato Porridge

Serving: 5

Prep Time: 10 minutes

Cook Time: 8 hours

**Ingredients:**

6 sweet potatoes, peeled and cut into 1-inch cubes

1 ½ cups light coconut milk

1 teaspoon ground cinnamon

1 teaspoon ground cardamom

1 teaspoon pure vanilla extract

1 cup raisins Pinch of salt

**How To:**

1. Add sweet potatoes coconut milk, vanilla, cardamom, cinnamon to your Slow Cooker.

2. Close lid and cook on LOW for 8 hours.

3. Open the lid and mash the entire mixture using potato masher to mash the sweet potatoes, stir well.

4. Stir in raisins, salt and serve.

5. Serve and enjoy!

## Nutrition (Per Serving)

Calories: 317

Fat: 4g

Carbohydrates: 71g

Protein: 4g

# A Nice German Oatmeal

Serving: 3

Prep Time: 10 minutes

Cook Time: 8 hours

**Ingredients:**

1 cup steel-cut oats

3 cups water

6 ounces coconut milk

2 tablespoons cocoa powder

1 tablespoon brown sugar

1 tablespoon coconut, shredded

**How to**

1. Grease the Slow Cooker well.
2. Add the listed ingredients to your Cooker and stir.
3. Place lid and cook on LOW for 8 hours.
4. Divide amongst serving bowls and enjoy!

**Nutrition (Per Serving)**

Calories: 200

Fat: 4g

Carbohydrates: 11g

Protein: 5g

# Very Nutty Banana Oatmeal

Serving: 4

Prep Time: 15 minutes

Cook Time: 7-9 hours

**Ingredients:**

1 cup steel-cut oats

1 ripe banana, mashed

2 cups unsweetened almond milk

1 cup water

1 ½ tablespoons honey

½ teaspoon vanilla extract

¼ cup almonds, chopped

1 teaspoon ground cinnamon

¼ teaspoon ground nutmeg

**How To:**

1. Grease the Slow Cooker well.

2. Add the listed ingredients to your Slow Cooker and stir.

3. Cover with lid and cook on LOW for 7-9 hours.

4. Serve and enjoy!

**Nutrition (Per Serving)**

Calories: 230

Fat: 7g

Carbohydrates: 40g

Protein: 5g

# Cool Coconut Flatbread

Serving: 4

Prep Time: 15 minutes

Cooking Time: 10 minutes

**Ingredients:**

1 ½ tablespoons coconut flour

¼ teaspoon baking powder

1/8 teaspoon sunflower seeds

1 tablespoon coconut oil, melted

1 whole egg

**How To:**

1. Preheat your oven to 350 degrees F.
2. Add coconut flour, leaven , sunflower seeds.
3. Add copra oil , eggs and stir well until mixed.
4. Leave the batter for several minutes.
5. Pour half the batter onto the baking pan.

6. Spread it to make a circle, repeat with remaining batter.

7. Bake within the oven for 10 minutes.

8. Once you get a golden-brown texture, let it cool and serve.

9. Enjoy!

**Nutrition (Per Serving)**

Total Carbs: 9 (%)

Fiber: 3g

Protein: 8g (%)

Fat: 20g (%)

# Perfect Homemade Pickled Ginger Gari

Serving: 8

Prep Time: 40 minutes

Cook Time: 5 minutes

**Ingredients:**

About 8 ounces of fresh ginger root, completely peeled

1 teaspoon and extra ½ teaspoon of fine sunflower seeds

1 cup vinegar, rice

1/3 cup sugar, white

**How To:**

1. Cut your ginger into small-sized chunks and transfer them to a bowl.

2. Season with sunflower seeds and stir, let the mixture sit for a minimum of half-hour .

3. Take a saucepan and add sugar and vinegar, heat it up, bring the mixture to a boil and keep boiling until the sugar has completely dissolved.

4. Pour the liquid over your ginger pieces.

5. Let it cool and wait until the water changes color.

6. Enjoy!

7. Alternatively, store in jars and use as required.

**Nutrition (Per Serving)**

Calories: 14

Fat: 0.1g

Carbohydrates: 3g

Protein: 0.1g

# Avocado and Blueberry Medley

Serving: 4

Prep Time: 5 minutes

Cook Time: Nil

**Ingredients:**

1 frozen banana

2 avocados, quartered

2 cups berries

Maple syrup as needed

**How To:**

1. Take your blender and add all ingredients except syrup.
2. Add drinking water and blend.
3. Garnish with syrup and pour in smoothie glasses.
4. Enjoy!

**Nutrition (Per Serving)**

Calories: 250

Fat: 13g

Carbohydrates: 40g

Protein 4g

# Healthy Zucchini Stir Fry

Serving: 4

Prep Time: 10 minutes

Cook Time: 10 minutes

**Ingredients:**

2 heaped tablespoons olive oil

1 medium-sized onion, sliced thinly

2 medium-sized zucchini, cut up into thin sized strips

2 heaped tablespoons teriyaki flavored sauce, low sodium

1 tablespoon coconut aminos

1 tablespoon sesame seed, toasted Ground pepper (black) as much as needed

**How To:**

1. Take a skillet and place it over medium level heat.
2. Add onions, and stir-cook for five minutes.
3. Add your zucchini and stir-cook for 1 minute more.

4. Gently add the sauces alongside the sesame seeds.

5. Cook for five minutes more until the zucchini are soft.

6. Finally, add the pepper and enjoy!

**Nutrition (Per Serving)**

Calories: 110

Fat: 9g

Carbohydrates: 8g

Protein: 3g

# Greek Lemon Chicken Bowl

Serving: 6

Prep Time: 10 minutes

Cook Time: 15 minutes

**Ingredients:**

2 cups chicken, cooked and chopped

2 cans chicken broth, fat free

2 medium carrots, chopped

¼ teaspoon pepper

2 tablespoons parsley, snipped

¼ cup lemon juice

1 can cream chicken soup, fat free, low sodium ½ cup onion, chopped

1 garlic clove, minced

**How To:**

1. Take a pot and add all the ingredients except parsley into it.

2. Season with salt and pepper.

3. Bring the combination to a overboil medium-high heat.

4. Reduce the warmth and simmer for quarter-hour .

5. Garnish with parsley.

6. Serve hot and enjoy!

**Nutrition (Per Serving)**

Calories: 520

Fat: 33g

Carbohydrates: 31g

Protein: 30g

# Chilled Chicken, Artichoke and Zucchini Platter

Serving: 4

Prep Time: 10 minutes

Cook Time: 5 minutes

**Ingredients:**

2 medium chicken breasts, cooked and cut into 1-inch cubes ¼ cup extra virgin olive oil

2 cups artichoke hearts, drained and roughly chopped

3 large zucchini, diced/cut into small rounds

1 can (15 ounce) chickpeas

1 cup Kalamata olives

½ teaspoon Fresh ground black pepper

½ teaspoon Italian seasoning

¼ cup parmesan, grated

**How To:**

1. Take an outsized skillet and place it over medium heat, heat up vegetable oil.

2. Add zucchini and sauté for five minutes, season with salt and pepper.

3. Remove from heat and add all the listed ingredients to the skillet.

4. Stir until combined.

5. Transfer to glass container and store.

6. Serve and enjoy!

**Nutrition (Per Serving)**

Calories: 457

Fat: 22g

Carbohydrates: 30g

Protein: 24g

# Chicken and Carrot Stew

Serving: 6

Prep Time: 15 minutes

Cook Time: 6 hours

**Ingredients:**

4 chicken breasts, boneless and cubed

2 cups chicken broth

1 cup tomatoes, chopped

3 cups carrots, peeled and cubed

1 teaspoon thyme dried

1 cup onion, chopped

2 garlic cloves, minced

Pepper to taste

**How To:**

1. Add all the ingredients to the Slow Cooker.
2. Stir and shut the lid.

3. Cook for six hours.

4. Serve hot and enjoy!

**Nutrition (Per Serving)**

Calories: 182

Fat: 4g

Carbohydrates: 10g

Protein: 39g

# Tasty Spinach Pie

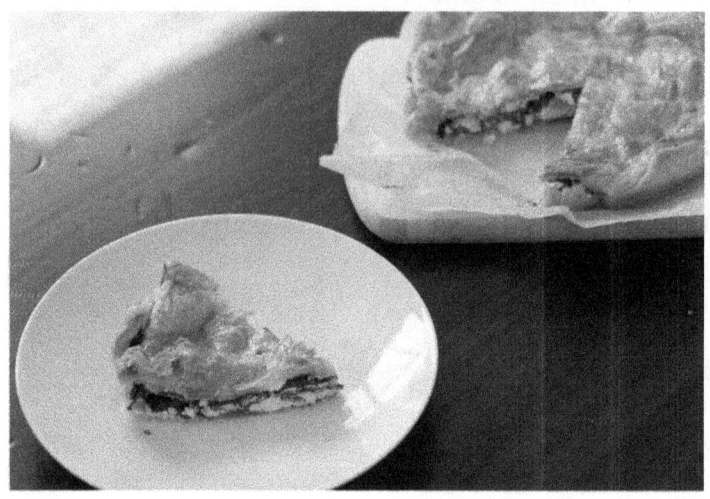

Serving: 2

Prep Time: 10 minutes

Cooking Time: 4 hours

## Ingredients:

10 ounces spinach

2 cups baby Bella mushrooms, chopped

1 red bell pepper, chopped

1 ½ cups low-fat cheese, shredded

8 whole eggs

1 cup coconut cream

2 tablespoons chives, chopped

Pinch of pepper

½ cup almond flour

¼ teaspoon baking soda

**How To:**

1. Take a bowl and add eggs, coconut milk , chives, pepper and whisk well.

2. Add almond flour, bicarbonate of soda , cheese, mushrooms bell pepper, spinach and toss well.

3. Grease your cooker and transfer mix to the Slow Cooker.

4. Place lid and cook on LOW for 4 hours.

5. Slice and enjoy!

**Nutrition (Per Serving)**

Calories: 201

Fat: 6g

Carbohydrates: 8g

Protein: 5g

# Mesmerizing Carrot and Pineapple Mix

Serving: 10

Prep Time: 10 minutes

Cooking Time: 6 hours

**Ingredients:**

1 cup raisins 6 cups water

23 ounces natural applesauce

2 tablespoons stevia

2 tablespoons cinnamon powder

14 ounces carrots, shredded

8 ounces canned pineapple, crushed

1 tablespoon pumpkin pie spice

**How To:**

1. Add carrots, applesauce, raisins, stevia, cinnamon, pineapple, pie spice to your Slow Cooker and gently stir.

2. Place lid and cook on LOW for six hours.

3. Serve and enjoy!

**Nutrition (Per Serving)**

Calories: 179

Fat: 5g

Carbohydrates: 15g

Protein: 4g

# Ethiopian Cabbage Delight

Serving: 6

Prep Time: 15 minutes

Cook Time: 6- 8 hours

**Ingredients:**

½ cup water

1 head green cabbage, cored and chopped

1-pound sweet potatoes, peeled and chopped

3 carrots, peeled and chopped

1 onion, sliced

1 teaspoon extra virgin olive oil

½ teaspoon ground turmeric

½ teaspoon ground cumin

¼ teaspoon ground ginger

**How To:**

1. Add water to your Slow Cooker.

2. Take a medium bowl and add cabbage, carrots, sweet potatoes, onion and blend.

3. Add vegetable oil, turmeric, ginger, cumin and toss until the veggies are fully coated.

4. Transfer veggie mix to your Slow Cooker.

5. Cover and cook on LOW for 6-8 hours.

6. Serve and enjoy!

**Nutrition (Per Serving)**

Calories: 155

Fat: 2g

Carbohydrates: 35g

Protein: 4g

# The Vegan Lovers Refried Beans

Serving: 12

Prep Time: 5 minutes

Cook Time: 10 hours

**Ingredients:**

4 cups vegetable broth

4 cups water

3 cups dried pinto beans

1 onion, chopped

2 jalapeno peppers, minced

4 garlic cloves, minced

1 tablespoon chili powder

2 teaspoon ground cumin

1 teaspoon sweet paprika

1 teaspoon salt

½ teaspoon fresh ground black pepper

**How To:**

1. Add the listed ingredients to your Slow Cooker.

2. Cover and cook on HIGH for 10 hours.

3. If there's any extra liquid, ladle the liquid up and reserve it during a bowl.

4. Use an immersion blender to blend the mixture (in the Slow Cooker) until smooth.

5. Add the reserved liquid.

6. Serve hot and enjoy!

**Nutrition (Per Serving)**

Calories: 91

Fat: 0g

Carbohydrates: 16g

Protein: 5g

# Cool Apple and Carrot Harmony

Serving: 6

Prep Time: 10 minutes

Cook Time: 10 minutes

**Ingredients:**

1 cup apple juice

1 pound baby carrots

1 tablespoon cornstarch

1 tablespoon mint, chopped

**How To:**

1. Add fruit juice, carrots, cornstarch and mint to your Instant Pot.
2. Stir and lock the lid.
3. Cook on high for 10 minutes.
4. Perform a fast release.
5. Divide the combination amongst plates and serve.

6. Enjoy!

## Nutrition (Per Serving)

Calories: 161

Fat: 2g

Carbohydrates: 9g

Protein: 8g

# Mac and Chokes

Serving: 6

Prep Time: 5 minutes

Cook Time: 20 minutes

**Ingredients:**

1 tablespoon of olive oil

1 large sized diced onion

10 minced garlic cloves

1 can artichoke hearts

1-pound uncooked macaroni shells

12-ounce baby spinach

4 cups vegetable broth

1 teaspoon red pepper flakes

4 ounces vegan cheese

¼ cup cashew cream

**How To:**

1. Set the pot to Sauté mode and add oil, allow the oil to heat up and add onions.

2. Cook for two minutes.

3. Add garlic and stir well.

4. Add artichoke hearts and sauté for 1 minute more.

5. Add uncooked pasta and three cups of broth alongside 2 cups of water.

6. Mix well.

7. Lock the lid and cook on high for 4 minutes.

8. Quick release the pressure.

9. Open the pot and stir.

10. Add extra water, fold in spinach and cook on Sauté mode for a couple of minutes.

11. Add cashew cream and grated vegan cheese.

12. Add pepper flakes and blend well.

13. Enjoy!

**Nutrition (Per Serving)**

Calories: 649

Fat: 29g

Carbohydrates: 64g

Protein: 34g

# Bay Scallop Chowder

Serving: 4

Prep Time: 10 minutes

Cook Time: 18 minutes

**Ingredients:**

1 medium onion, chopped

2 ½ cups chicken stock

4 slices bacon, chopped

3 cups daikon radish, chopped

½ teaspoon dried thyme

2 cups low-fat cream

1 tablespoon almond butter

Pepper to taste

1 pound bay scallops

**How To:**

1. Heat olive over medium heat in a large sized saucepan, add bacon and cook until crisp, add onion and daikon radish.

2. Cook for 5 minutes, add chicken stock.

3. Simmer for 8 minutes, season with salt and pepper, thyme.

4. Add heavy cream, bay scallops, simmer for 4 minutes

5.    Serve and enjoy!

**Nutrition (Per Serving)**

Calories: 307

Fat: 22g

Carbohydrates: 7g

Protein: 22g

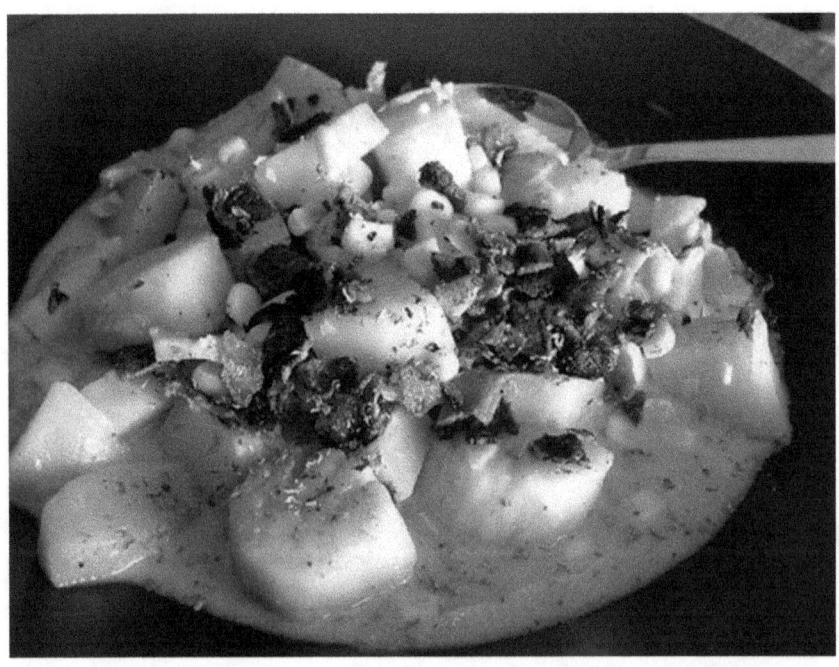

# Salmon and Vegetable Soup

Serving: 4

Prep Time: 10 minutes

Cook Time: 22 minutes

**Ingredients:**

2 tablespoons extra-virgin olive oil

1 leek, chopped

1 red onion, chopped

Pepper to taste

2 carrots, chopped

4 cups low stock vegetable stock

4 ounces salmon, skinless and boneless, cubed ½ cup coconut cream

1 tablespoon dill, chopped

**How To:**

1. Take a pan and place it over medium heat, add leek, onion, stir and cook for 7 minutes.

2. Add pepper, carrots, stock and stir.

3. Boil for 10 minutes.

4. Add salmon, cream, dill and stir.

5. Boil for 5-6 minutes.
6. Ladle into bowls and serve.
7. Enjoy!

**Nutrition (Per Serving)**

Calories: 240

Fat: 4g

Carbohydrates: 7g

Protein: 12g

# Garlic Tomato Soup

Serving: 4

Prep Time: 15 minutes

Cook Time: 15 minutes

**Ingredients:**

Roma tomatoes, chopped

1 cup tomatoes, sundried

2 tablespoons coconut oil

5 garlic cloves, chopped

14 ounces coconut milk

1 cup vegetable broth

Pepper to taste

Basil, for garnish

**How To:**

1. Take a pot, heat oil into it.
2. Sauté the garlic in it for ½ minute.
3. Mix in the Roma tomatoes and cook for 8-10 minutes.
4. Stir occasionally.
5. Add in the rest of the ingredients, except the basil, and stir well.

6. Cover the lid and cook for 5 minutes.

7. Let it cool.

8. Blend the soup until smooth by using an immersion blender.

9. Garnish with basil.

10. Serve and enjoy!

**Nutrition (Per Serving)**

Calories: 240

Fat: 23g

Carbohydrates: 16g

Protein: 7g

# Melon Soup

Serving: 4

Prep Time: 6 minutes

Cook Time: Nil

## Ingredients:

4 cups casaba melon, seeded and cubed

1 tablespoon fresh ginger, grated

¾ cup coconut milk Juice of 2 limes

## How To:

Add the lime juice, coconut milk, casaba melon, ginger and salt into your blender.

Blend for 1-2 minutes until you get a smooth mixture.

Serve and enjoy!

## Nutrition (Per Serving)

Calories: 134

Fat: 9g

Carbohydrates: 13g

Protein: 2g

# Spring Salad

Serving: 2

Prep Time: 10-15 minutes

Cook Time: 0 minutes

## Ingredients:

2 ounces mixed green vegetables

3 tablespoons roasted pine nuts

2 tablespoons 5-minute 5 Keto Raspberry Vinaigrette

2 tablespoons shaved Parmesan

2 slices bacon

Pepper as required

## How To:

1. Take a cooking pan and add bacon, cook the bacon until crispy.

2. Take a bowl and add the salad ingredients and mix well, add crumbled bacon into the salad.

3. Mix well.

4. Dress it with your favorite dressing.

5. Enjoy!

**Nutrition (Per Serving)**

Calories: 209

Fat: 17g

Net Carbohydrates: 10g

Protein: 4g

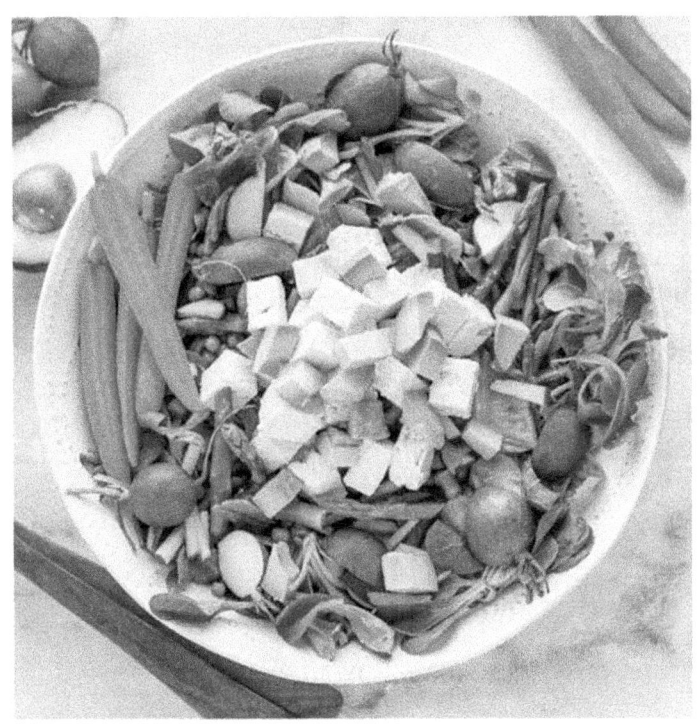

# Hearty Orange and Onion Salad

Serving: 2

Prep Time: 10 minutes

Cook Time: nil

**Ingredients:**

6 large oranges

3 tablespoons red wine vinegar

6 tablespoons olive oil

1 teaspoon dried oregano

1 red onion, thinly sliced

1 cup olive oil

¼ cup fresh chives, chopped Ground black pepper

**How To:**

1. Peel orange and cut into 4-5 crosswise slices.
2. Transfer orange to shallow dish.
3. Drizzle vinegar, olive oil on top.
4. Sprinkle oregano.
5. Toss well to mix.
6. Chill for 30 minutes and arrange sliced onion and black olives on top.

7. Sprinkle more chives and pepper.

8. Serve and enjoy!

## Nutrition (Per Serving)

Calories: 120

Fat: 6g

Carbohydrates: 20g

Protein: 2g

# Ground Beef Bell Peppers

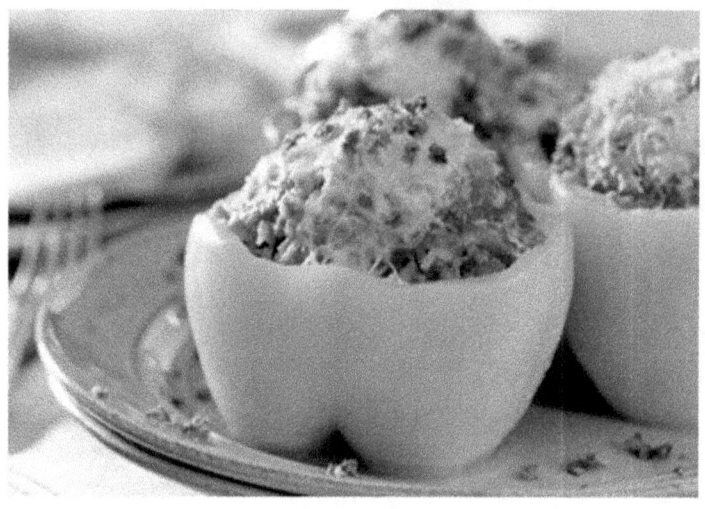

Serving: 3

Prep Time: 10 minutes

Cook Time: 10 minutes

**Ingredients:**

1 onion, chopped

2 tablespoons coconut oil

1 pound ground beef

1 red bell pepper, diced

2 cups spinach, chopped

Pepper to taste

**How To:**

1. Take a skillet and place it over medium heat.
2. Add onion and cook until slightly browned.
3. Add spinach and ground beef.
4. Stir fry until done.
5. Take the mixture and fill up the bell peppers.
6. Serve and enjoy!

**Nutrition (Per Serving)**

Calories: 350

Fat: 23g

Carbohydrates: 4g

Protein: 28g

# Ecstatic "Foiled" Fish

Serving: 4

Prep Time: 20 minutes

Cook Time: 40 minutes

**Ingredients:**

2 rainbow trout fillets

tablespoon olive oil

teaspoon garlic salt

1 teaspoon ground black pepper

1 fresh jalapeno pepper, sliced

1 lemon, sliced

**How To:**

1. Pre-heat your oven to 400 degrees F.
2. Rinse your fish and pat them dry.
3. Rub the fillets with olive oil, season with some garlic salt and black pepper.

4. Place each of your seasoned fillets on a large sized sheet of aluminum foil.

5. Top it with some jalapeno slices and squeeze the juice from your lemons over your fish.

6. Arrange the lemon slices on top of your fillets.

7. Carefully seal up the edges of your foil and form a nice enclosed packet.

8. Place your packets on your baking sheet.

9. Bake them for about 20 minutes.

10. Once the flakes start to flake off with a fork, the fish is ready!

**Nutrition (Per Serving)**

Calories: 213

Fat: 10g

Carbohydrates: 8g

Protein: 24g

# Brazilian Shrimp Stew

Serving: 4

Prep Time: 20 minutes

Cook Time: 25 minutes

**Ingredients:**

Tablespoons lime juice

1 ½ tablespoons cumin, ground

½ tablespoons paprika

½ teaspoons garlic, minced

½ teaspoons pepper

Pounds tilapia fillets, cut into bits

1 large onion, chopped

Large bell peppers, cut into strips

1 can (14 ounces) tomato, drained

1 can (14 ounces) coconut milk handful of cilantros, chopped

**How To:**

1. Take a large sized bowl and add lime juice, cumin, paprika, garlic, pepper and mix well.
2. Add tilapia and coat it up.
3. Cover and allow to marinate for 20 minutes.
4. Set your Instant Pot to Sauté mode and add olive oil.
5. Add onions and cook for 3 minutes until tender.
6. Add pepper strips, tilapia, and tomatoes to a skillet.
7. Pour coconut milk and cover, simmer for 20 minutes.
8. Add cilantro during the final few minutes.
9. Serve and enjoy!

**Nutrition (Per Serving)**

Calories: 471

Fat: 44g

Carbohydrates: 13g

Protein: 12g

# Inspiring Cajun Snow Crab

Serving: 2

Prep Time: 10 minutes

Cook Time: 10 minutes

## Ingredients:

1 lemon, fresh and quartered tablespoons

Cajun seasoning

Bay leaves

Snow crab legs, precooked and defrosted Golden ghee

## How To:

1. Take a large pot and fill it about halfway with sunflower seeds and water.

2. Bring the water to a boil.

3. Squeeze lemon juice into the pot and toss in remaining lemon quarters.

4. Add bay leaves and Cajun seasoning.

5. Season for 1 minute.

6.   Add crab legs and boil for 8 minutes (make sure to keep them submerged the whole time).

7.   Melt ghee in microwave and use as dipping sauce, enjoy!

**Nutrition (Per Serving)**

Calories: 643

Fat: 51g

Carbohydrates: 3g

Protein: 41g

# Grilled Lime Shrimp

Serving: 8

Prep Time: 25 minutes

Cook Time: 5 minutes

**Ingredients:**

1-pound medium shrimp, peeled and deveined

1 lime, juiced

½ cup olive oil

Cajun seasoning

**How To:**

1. Take a re-sealable zip bag and add lime juice, Cajun seasoning, olive oil.

2. Add shrimp and shake it well, let it marinate for 20 minutes.

3. Pre-heat your outdoor grill to medium heat.

4. Lightly grease the grate.

5. Remove shrimp from marinade and cook for 2 minutes per side.

6. Serve and enjoy!

**Nutrition (Per Serving)**

Calories: 188

Fat: 3g

Net Carbohydrates: 1.2g

Protein: 13g

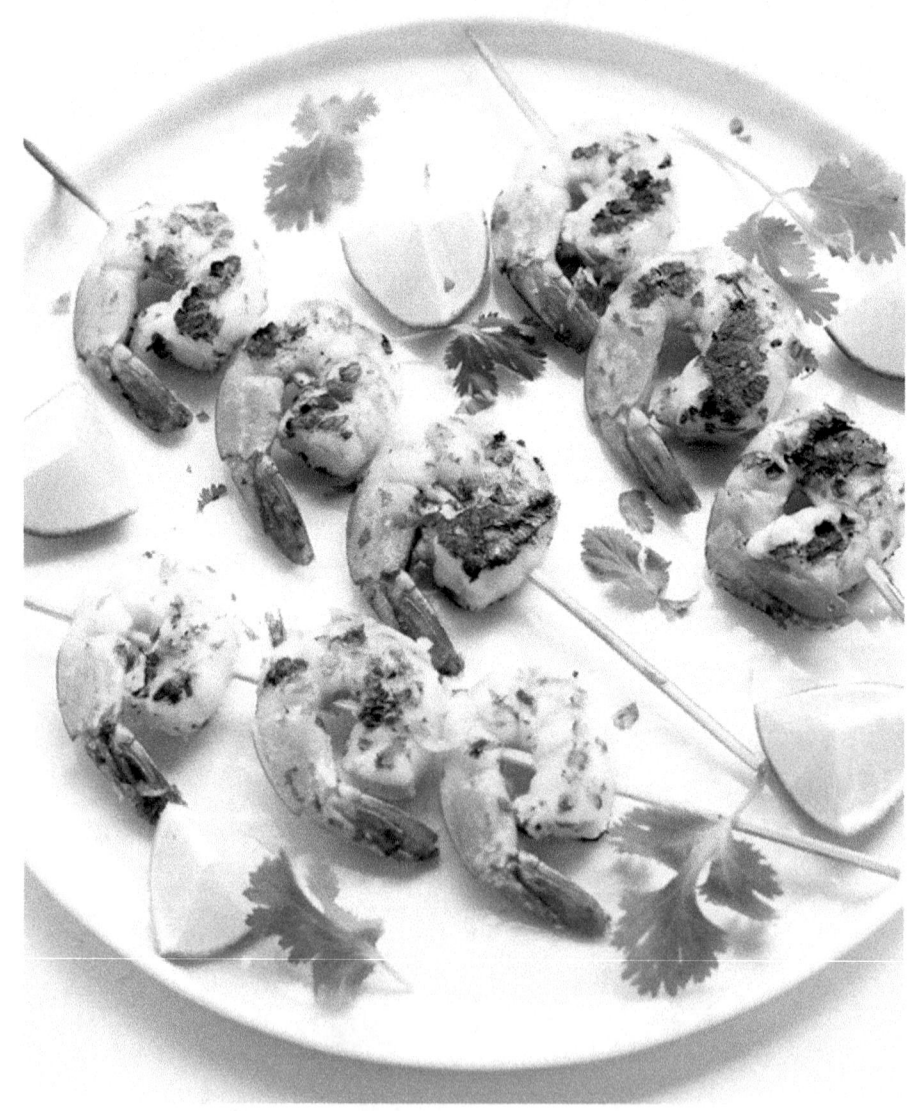

# Calamari Citrus

Serving: 4

Prep Time: 10 minutes

Cook Time: 5 minutes

**Ingredients:**

1 lime, sliced

lemon, sliced

Pounds calamari tubes and tentacles, sliced

Pepper to taste

¼ cup olive oil

garlic cloves, minced

tablespoons lemon juice

orange, peeled and cut into segments

tablespoons cilantro, chopped

**How To:**

1. Take a bowl and add calamari, pepper, lime slices, lemon slices, orange slices, garlic, oil, cilantro, lemon juice and toss well.

2. Take a pan and place it over medium-high heat.

3. Add calamari mix and cook for 5 minutes.

4. Divide into bowls and serve.

5. Enjoy!

**Nutrition (Per Serving)**

Calories: 190

Fat: 2g

Net Carbohydrates: 11g

Protein: 14g

# Baked Chicken

Prep time: 10 minutes

Cook time: 1 hour

Servings: 4

## Ingredients

Chicken – 3 to 4 pounds, cut into parts Olive oil – 3 Tbsp.

Thyme – ½ tsp.

Sea salt – ¼ tsp.

Ground black pepper

Low-sodium chicken stock – ½ cup

## Method

1.   Preheat the oven to 400F.

2.   Rub oil over chicken pieces. Sprinkle with salt, thyme, and pepper.

3.   Place chicken in the roasting pan.

4.   Bake in the oven for 30 minutes.

5. Then lower the heat to 350F.

6. Bake for 15 to 30 minutes more or until juice runs clear.

7. Serve.

**Nutritional Facts Per Serving**

Calories: 550

Fat: 19g

Carb: 0g

Protein: 91g

Sodium 480mg

# Orange Chicken and Broccoli Stir-Fry

Prep time: 10 minutes

Cook time: 15 minutes

Servings: 4

**Ingredients**

Olive oil – 1 Tbsp.

Chicken breast – 1 pound, boneless and skinless, cut into strips
Orange juice – 1/3 cup Homemade soy sauce - 2 Tbsp.

Cornstarch – 2 tsp.

Broccoli – 2 cups, cut into small pieces Snow peas – 1 cup

Cabbage – 2 cups, shredded Brown rice – 2 cups, cooked
Sesame seeds – 1 Tbsp.

**Method**

1. Combine the orange juice, soy sauce, and corn starch in a bowl. Set aside.

2. Heat oil in a pan. Add chicken.

3.  Stir-fry until the chicken is golden brown on all sides, about 5 minutes.

4.  Add snow peas, cabbage, broccoli, and sauce mixture.

5.  Continue to stir-fry for 8 minutes or until vegetables are tender but still crisp.

**Nutritional Facts Per Serving**

Calories: 340

Fat: 8g

Carb: 35g

Protein: 28g

Sodium 240mg

# Mediterranean Lemon Chicken and Potatoes

Prep time: 10 minutes

Cook time: 30 minutes

Servings: 4

**Ingredients**

Chicken breast – 1 ½ pound, skinless and boneless, cut into 1-inch cubes

Yukon Gold potatoes – 1 pound, cut into cubes

Onion – 1, chopped

Red pepper – 1, chopped

Low-sodium vinaigrette – ½ cup

Lemon juice – ¼ cup Oregano – 1 tsp.

Garlic powder – ½ tsp.

Chopped tomato – ½ cup

Ground black pepper to taste

## Method

1. Preheat oven to 400F.

2. Except for the tomatoes, mix everything in a bowl.

3. On 4 aluminum foils, place an equal amount of chicken and potato mixture. Fold to make packets.

4. Bake at 400F for 30 minutes. Open packets.

5. Top with chopped tomatoes.

6. Season with black pepper to taste.

## Nutritional Facts Per Serving

Calories: 320

Fat: 4g

Carb: 34g

Protein: 43g

Sodium 420mg

# Tandoori Chicken

Prep time: 10 minutes

Cook time: 20 minutes

Servings: 6

**Ingredients**

Nonfat yogurt – 1 cup, plain

Lemon juice – ½ cup Garlic – 5 cloves, crushed Paprika – 2 Tbsp.

Curry powder – 1 tsp.

Ground ginger – 1 tsp.

Red pepper flakes – 1 tsp.

Chicken breasts – 6, skinless and boneless, cut into 2-inch chunks Wooden skewers – 6, soaked in water

**Method**

1. Preheat the oven to 400F.

2. In a bowl, combine lemon juice, yogurt, garlic, and spices. Blend well.

3.	Divide chicken and thread onto skewers. Place skewers in a baking dish.

4.	Pour half of the yogurt mixture onto chicken. Cover and marinate in the refrigerator for 20 minutes

5.	Spray a baking dish with cooking spray.

6.	Place chicken skewers in the pan and coat with the remaining ½ of yogurt marinade.

7.	Bake in the oven until chicken is cooked, about 15 to 20 minutes.

8.	Serve with veggies or brown rice.

**Nutritional Facts Per Serving**

Calories: 175

Fat: 2g

Carb: 8g

Protein: 30g

Sodium 105mg

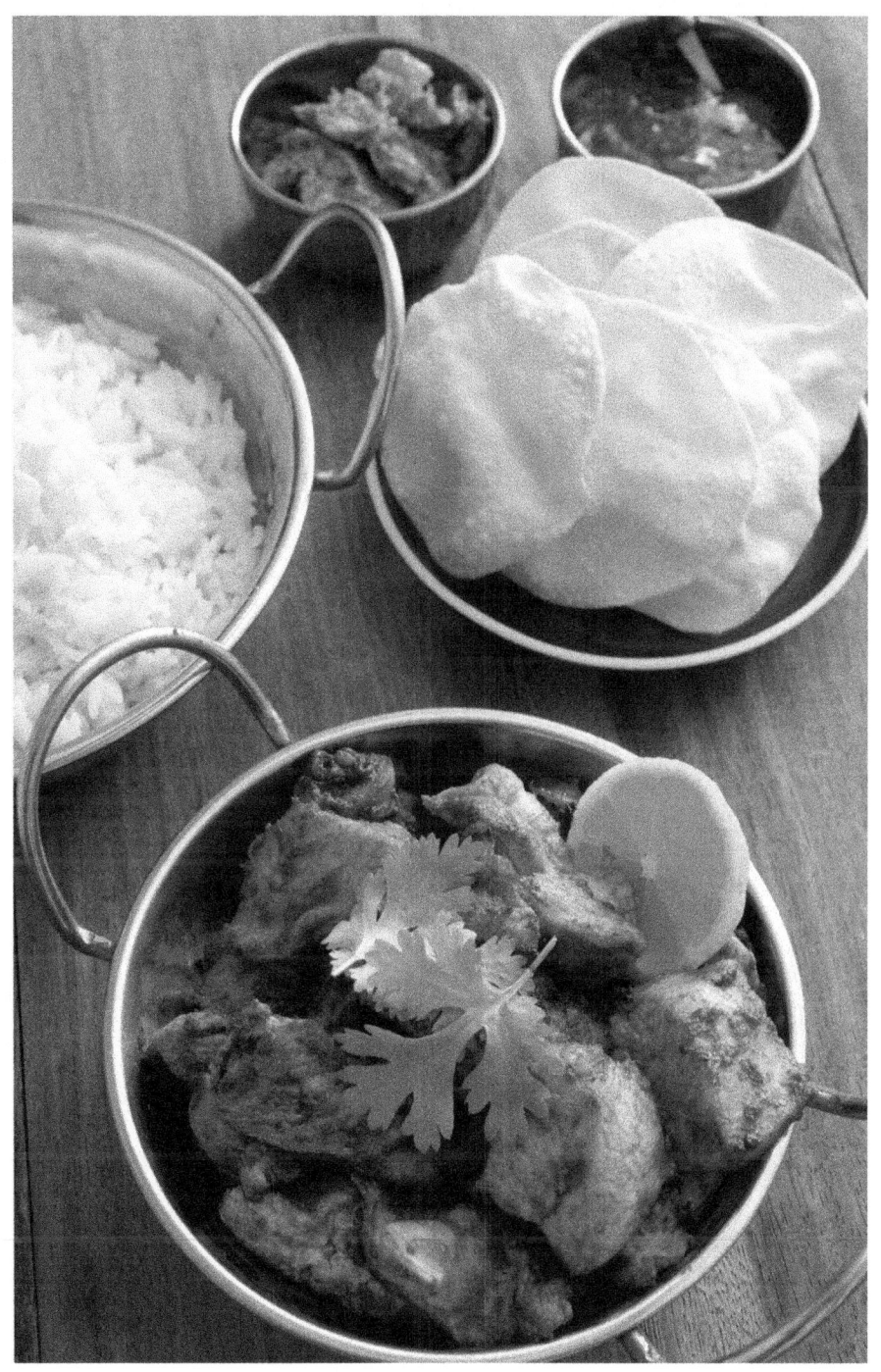

# Grilled Chicken Salad

Prep time: 5 minutes

Cook time: 10 minutes

Servings: 4

**Ingredients**

For the dressing

Red wine vinegar – ½ cup

Garlic – 4 cloves, minced

Extra-virgin olive oil – 1 Tbsp.

Finely chopped red onion – 1 Tbsp.

Finely chopped celery -1 Tbsp. Ground black pepper to taste For the salad

Chicken breasts – 4 (4-ounce each), boneless, skinless

Garlic – 2 cloves

Lettuce leaves - 8 cups

Ripe black olives – 16

Navel oranges – 2, peeled and sliced

## Method

1. To make the dressing, in a bowl, combine all the dressing ingredients mix and keep in the refrigerator.

2. Heat a gas grill or broiler.

3. Lightly coat the broiler pan or grill rack with cooking spray.

4. Position the cooking rack 4 to 6 inches from the heat source.

5. Rub the chicken breasts with garlic and discard the cloves.

6. Broil or grill the chicken about 5 minutes per side, or until just cooked through.

7. Slice the chicken. Arrange with lettuce, olives, and oranges.

8. Drizzle with dressing and serve.

## Nutritional Facts Per Serving

Calories: 237
Fat: 9g
Carb: 12g
Protein: 27g
Sodium 199mg

# Hearty Cashew and Almond Butter

Serving: 1 and ½ cups

Prep Time: 5 minutes

Cook Time: Nil

**Ingredients:**

1 cup almonds, blanched

1/3 cup cashew nuts

2 tablespoons coconut oil

½ teaspoon cinnamon

**How To:**

1. Pre-heat your oven to 350 degrees F.
2. Bake almonds and cashews for 12 minutes.
3. Let them cool.
4. Transfer to food processor and add remaining ingredients.
5. Add oil and keep blending until smooth.

6. Serve and enjoy!

**Nutrition (Per Serving)**

Calories: 205

Fat: 19g

Carbohydrates: g

Protein: 2.8g

# Red Coleslaw

Serving: 4

Prep Time: 10 minutes

Cook Time: 0 minutes

**Ingredients:**

1 2/3 pounds red cabbage

2 tablespoons ground caraway seeds

1 tablespoon whole grain mustard

1 1/4 cups mayonnaise, low fat, low sodium Salt and black pepper

**How To:**

1. Cut the red cabbage into small slices.
2. Take a large-sized bowl and add all the ingredients alongside cabbage.
3. Mix well, season with salt and pepper.
4. Serve and enjoy!

**Nutrition (Per Serving)**

Calories: 406

Fat: 40.8g

Carbohydrates: 10g

Protein: 2.2g

# Avocado Mayo Medley

Serving: 4

Prep Time: 5 minutes

Cook Time: Nil

**Ingredients:**

1 medium avocado, cut into chunks

½ teaspoon ground cayenne pepper

2 tablespoons fresh cilantro

¼ cup olive oil

½ cup mayo, low fat and los sodium

**How To:**

1. Take a food processor and add avocado, cayenne pepper, lime juice, salt and cilantro.

2. Mix until smooth.

3. Slowly incorporate olive oil, add 1 tablespoon at a time and keep processing between additions.

4. Store and use as needed!

**Nutrition (Per Serving)**

Calories: 231

Fat: 20g

Carbohydrates: 5g

Protein: 3g

# Amazing Garlic Aioli

Serving: 4

Prep Time: 5 minutes

Cook Time: Nil

**Ingredients:**

½ cup mayonnaise, low fat and low sodium 2 garlic cloves, minced Juice of 1 lemon

1 tablespoon fresh-flat leaf Italian parsley, chopped

1 teaspoon chives, chopped Salt and pepper to taste

**How To:**

1. Add mayonnaise, garlic, parsley, lemon juice, chives and season with salt and pepper.

2. Blend until combined well.

3. Pour into refrigerator and chill for 30 minutes.

4. Serve and use as needed!

**Nutrition (Per Serving)**

Calories: 813

Fat: 88g

Carbohydrates: 9g

Protein: 2g

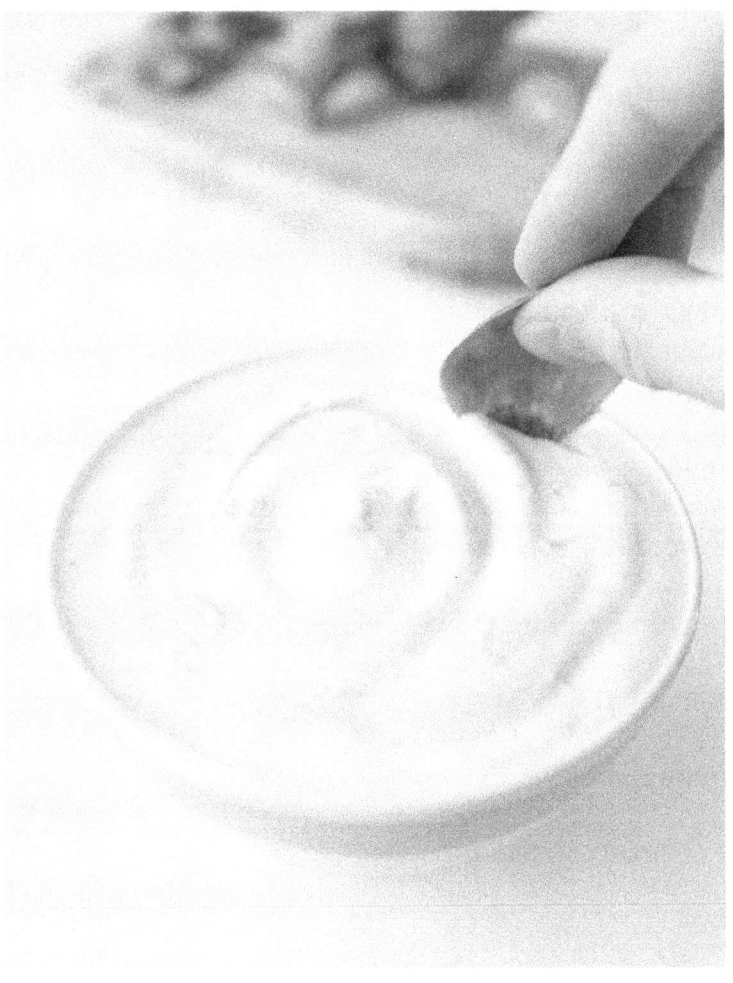

# Easy Seed Crackers

Serving: 72 crackers

Prep Time: 10 minutes

Cooking Time: 60 minutes

**Ingredients:**

1 cup boiling water

1/3 cup chia seeds

1/3 cup sesame seeds

1/3 cup pumpkin seeds

1/3 cup Flaxseeds

1/3 cup sunflower seeds

1 tablespoon Psyllium powder

1 cup almond flour

1 teaspoon salt

¼ cup coconut oil, melted

**How To:**

1. Pre-heat your oven to 300 degrees F.

2. Line a cookie sheet with parchment paper and keep it on the side.

3. Add listed ingredients (except coconut oil and water) to food processor and pulse until ground.

4. Transfer to a large mixing bowl and pour melted coconut oil and boiling water, mix.

5. Transfer mix to prepared sheet and spread into a thin layer.

6. Cut dough into crackers and bake for 60 minutes.

7. Cool and serve.

8. Enjoy!

**Nutrition (Per Serving)**

Total Carbs: 10.6g

Fiber: 3g

Protein: 5g

Fat: 14.6g

# Hearty Almond Crackers

Serving: 40 crackers

Prep Time: 10 minutes

Cooking Time: 20 minutes

**Ingredients:**

1 cup almond flour

¼ teaspoon baking soda

1/8 teaspoon black pepper

3 tablespoons sesame seeds

1 egg, beaten

Salt and pepper to taste

**How To:**

1. Pre-heat your oven to 350 degrees F.

2. Line two baking sheets with parchment paper and keep them on the side.

3. Mix the dry ingredients in a large bowl and add egg, mix well and form dough.

4. Divide dough into two balls.

5. Roll out the dough between two pieces of parchment paper.

6. Cut into crackers and transfer them to prepared baking sheet.

7. Bake for 15-20 minutes.

8. Repeat until all the dough has been used up.

9. Leave crackers to cool and serve.

10. Enjoy!

**Nutrition (Per Serving)**

Total Carbs: 8g

Fiber: 2g

Protein: 9g

Fat: 28g

# Black Bean Salsa

Serving: 4

Prep Time: 10 minutes

Cook Time: Nil

**Ingredients:**

1 tablespoon coconut amines

½ teaspoon cumin, ground

1 cup canned black beans, no salt

1 cup salsa

6 cups romaine lettuce, torn

½ cup avocado, peeled, pitted and cubed

**How To:**

1. Take a bowl and add beans, alongside other ingredients.
2. Toss well and serve.
3. Enjoy!

**Nutrition (Per Serving)**

Calories: 181

Fat: 5g

Carbohydrates: 14g

Protein: 7g

# Delish Pineapple and Coconut Milk Smoothie

Serving: 2

Prep Time: 5 minutes

**Ingredients:**

¼ cup pineapple, frozen

¾ cup coconut milk

**How To:**

1. Add the listed ingredients to blender and blend well on high.

2. Once the mixture is smooth, pour smoothie in tall glass and serve.

3. Chill and enjoy!

**Nutrition (Per Serving)**

Calories: 200

Fat: 10g

Carbohydrates: 14g

Protein 2g

# The Minty Refresher

Serving: 2

Prep Time: 5 minutes

**Ingredients:**

2 cups mint tea

1 cucumber, peeled

2 green apples

1 cup blueberries

Stevia (to sweeten)

Few slices of lime/lemon for garnish

**How To:**

1. Add the listed ingredients to your blender and blend until smooth.

2. Add ice and sweeten with a bit of stevia.

3. Garnish with lime/lemon slices.

4. Serve and enjoy!

**Nutrition (Per Serving)**

Calories: 200

Fat: 10g

Carbohydrates: 14g

Protein 2g

# The "Upbeat" Strawberry and Clementine Glass

Serving: 2

Prep Time: 5 minutes

**Ingredients:**

8 ounces strawberries, fresh

1 banana, chopped into chunks

2 Clementines/Mandarins

**How To:**

1. Peel the clementines and remove seeds.
2. Add the listed ingredients to your blender/food processor and blend until smooth.
3. Serve chilled and enjoy!

**Nutrition (Per Serving)**

Calories: 200

Fat: 10g

Carbohydrates: 14g

Protein 2g

# Cabbage and Coconut Chia Smoothie

Serving: 2

Prep Time: 5 minutes

**Ingredients:**

1/3 cup cabbage

1 cup cold unsweetened coconut milk

1 tablespoon chia seeds

½ cup cherries

½ cup spinach

**How To:**

1. Add coconut milk to your blender.
2. Cut cabbage and add to your blender.
3. Place chia seeds in a coffee grinder and chop to powder, brush the powder into the blender.
4. Pit the cherries and add them to the blender.
5. Wash and dry the spinach and chop.

6. Add to the mix.

7. Cover and blend on low followed by medium.

8. Taste the texture and serve chilled!

**Nutrition (Per Serving)**

Calories: 200

Fat: 10g

Carbohydrates: 14g

Protein 2g

# The Cherry Beet Delight

Serving: 2

Prep Time: 5 minutes

**Ingredients:**

1 cup cherries, pitted

½ cup beets

Few banana slices

1 cup water, filtered, alkaline

1 cup coconut milk

Pinch of organic vanilla powder

Pinch of cinnamon

Pinch of stevia

Few mint leaves/lime slices to garnish

**How To:**

1.   Add berries, beets, water, banana slices, coconut milk to your blender.

2. Blend well until smooth.

3. Add more water if the texture is too creamy for you.

4. Add coconut oil, vanilla, cinnamon and stir.

5. Add a bit of stevia for extra sweetness.

6. Garnish with mint leaves and lime slices.

7. Enjoy!

## Nutrition (Per Serving)

Calories: 200

Fat: 10g

Carbohydrates: 14g

Protein 2g

# Satisfying Honey and Coconut Porridge

Serving: 8

Prep Time: 10 minutes

Cook Time: 8 hours

**Ingredients:**

4 cups light coconut milk

3 cups apple juice

2 ¼ cups coconut flour

1 teaspoon ground cinnamon

¼ cup honey

**How To:**

1. In a Slow Cooker, add the coconut milk, apple juice, flour, cinnamon and honey.
2. Stir well.
3. Close lid and cook on LOW for 8 hours.
4. Open lid and stir.
5. Serve with an additional seasoning of fresh fruits.
6. Enjoy!

**Nutrition (Per Serving)**

Calories: 372

Fat: 14g

Carbohydrates: 56g

Protein: 8g

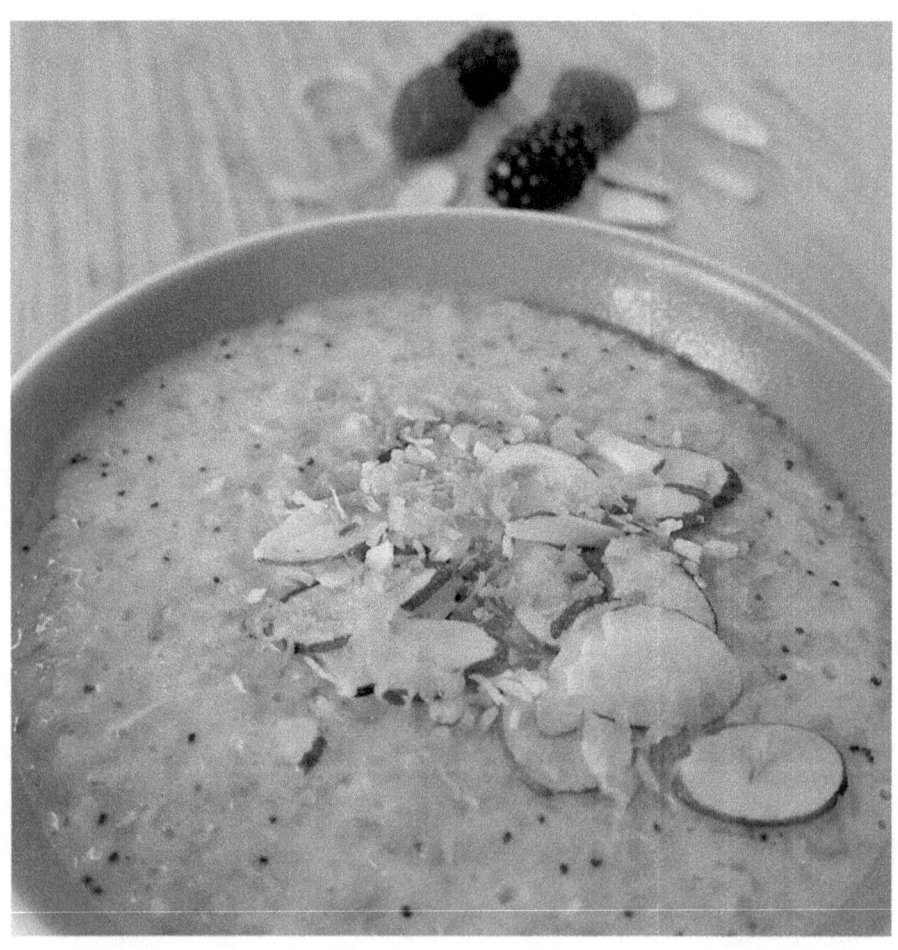

# Pure Maple Glazed Carrots

Serving: 6

Prep Time: 10 minutes

Cook Time: 8 hours

## Ingredients:

¼ cup pure maple syrup

½ teaspoon ground ginger

¼ teaspoon ground nutmeg

½ teaspoon salt

Juice of 1 orange

1-pound baby carrots

## How To:

1. Take a small bowl and whisk in syrup, nutmeg, ginger, salt, orange juice.

2. Add carrots to your Slow Cooker and pour the maple syrup.

3. Toss to coat.

4. Close lid and cook on LOW for 8 hours.

5. Serve and enjoy!

**Nutrition (Per Serving)**

Calories: 76

Fat: 1g

Carbohydrates: 19g

Protein: 76g

# Ginger and Orange "Beets"

Serving: 6

Prep Time: 20 minutes

Cook Time: 8 hours

## Ingredients:

2 pounds beets, peeled and cut into wedges

Juice of 2 oranges

Zest of 1 orange

1 teaspoon fresh ginger, grated

1 tablespoon honey

1 tablespoon apple cider vinegar

1/8 teaspoon fresh ground black pepper Sea salt

## How To:

1. Add beets, zest, orange juice, ginger, honey, pepper, salt and vinegar to your Slow Cooker.

2. Stir well.

3. Close lid and cook on LOW for 8 hours.

4. Serve and enjoy!

**Nutrition (Per Serving)**

Calories: 108

Fat: 1g

Carbohydrates: 25g

Protein: 3g

# Pineapple Rice

Serving: 2

Prep Time: 10 minutes

Cook Time: 2 hours

**Ingredients:**

1 cup rice

2 cups water

1 small cauliflower, florets separated and chopped ½ small pineapple, peeled and chopped Salt and pepper as needed

1 teaspoon olive oil

**How To:**

1. Add rice, cauliflower, pineapple, water, oil, salt and pepper to your Slow Cooker.
2. Gently stir.
3. Place lid and cook on HIGH for 2 hours.
4. Fluff the rice with fork and season with more salt and pepper if needed.
5. Divide between serving platters and enjoy!

**Nutrition (Per Serving)**

Calories: 152

Fat: 4g

Carbohydrates: 18g

Protein: 4g

# Creative Lemon and Broccoli Dish

Serving: 6

Prep Time: 10 minutes

Cook Time: 15 minutes

**Ingredients:**

2 heads broccoli, separated into florets

2 teaspoons extra virgin olive oil

1 teaspoon sunflower seeds

½ teaspoon black pepper

1 garlic clove, minced

½ teaspoon lemon juice

How To:

1. Pre-heat your oven to 400 degrees F.
2. Take a large sized bowl and add broccoli florets.
3. Drizzle olive oil and season with pepper, sunflower seeds and garlic.
4. Spread broccoli out in a single even layer on a baking sheet.
5. Bake for 15-20 minutes until fork tender.
6. Squeeze lemon juice on top.

7. Serve and enjoy!

**Nutrition (Per Serving)**

Calories: 49

Fat: 1.9g

Carbohydrates: 7g

Protein: 3g

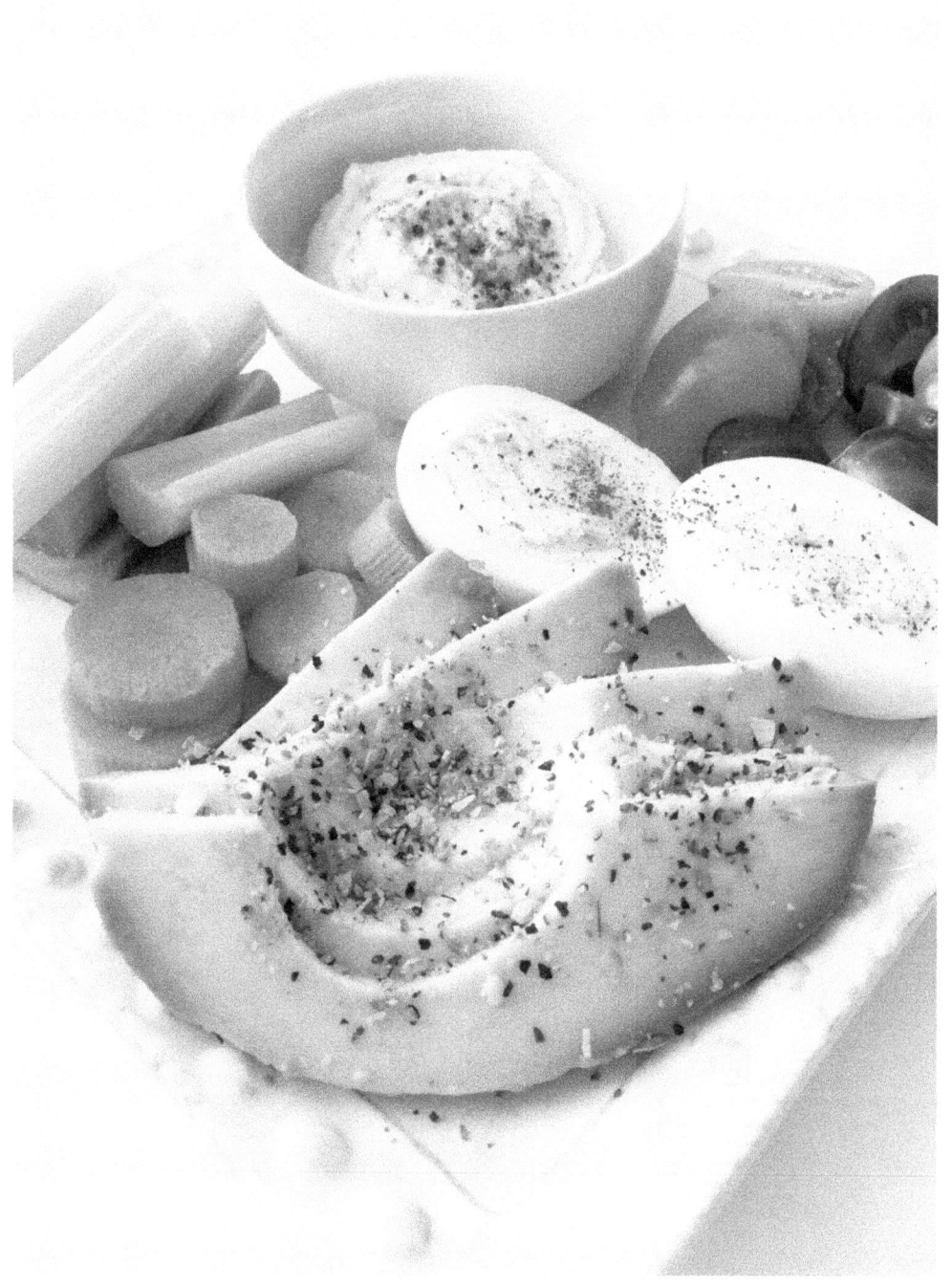

www.ingramcontent.com/pod-product-compliance
Lightning Source LLC
Chambersburg PA
CBHW071110030426
42336CB00013BA/2031